CARAN BOOKS

Alternative Medicine You Never Heard About

About
Part 2

Alternative medicine is separate from conventional medical approaches used in the United States. Alternative medical include homeopathic medicine and naturopathic medicine.

Louis Square

Disclaimer

Please note: This book is only for information purposes. This book is not intended to be medical advice and it is not a substitute for professional advice. Please consult your health professionals for your concerns. Please follow any tips given in this article only after consulting your medical doctor. The author is not liable for any outcome or damage resulting from information obtained from this book.

Introduction:

My wife and I have a close friend who is suffering from a very serious disease.

Being somewhat educated and totally clueless about non-traditional medical treatments we decided to do some research.

Utilizing the Internet we started researching Alternative Medicine. Wow! I was over whelmed by all the different views and opinions out there.

Along the way I found it difficult to locate centralized information about alternative treatments that was understandable. Not wishing others to have such a difficult time I decided to put all the important information in one place. That is how "Alternative Medicine You Never Heard About" was conceived.

I sincerely hope that you learn some useful facts that will help you to understand alternative treatments!

Louis Square

Ginkgo Biloba

Introduction:

Ginkgo trees, are one of the oldest species of trees cultivated in China and are believed to be 150 to 200 million years old. The ginkgo trees grow in average soil and even in full sun. The tree can grow 100 – 120 feet. Ginkgo trees are very resistant to pollution and infection and hardly suffer any disease. Insects rarely attack these plants. Due to these reasons these trees are most tolerant even in urban conditions and are grown as shade trees.

Ginkgo or ginkgo biloba extracts is made from various parts of these trees. Chinease has used ginkgo biloba for the centuries for treating various ailments. Now it is most researched herb and is used by most of the countries as herbal medicine.

Working of Ginkgo Biloba:

Ginkgo leaves contains two groups of active components known as flavonoid glycosides and ginkgolides. These active ingredients helps in increasing blood flow to the brain and improving overall network of blood vessels, and consequently increases the inflow of oxygen and essential nutrients to brain and other important organs of the body and simultaneously helps controlling in allergic inflammation and asthma.

Benefits of Ginkgo Biloba:

The research on this herbal medicine continues for the last three decades and some of the benefits as evidenced by clinical studies have been summarized below.

- It has a positive effect on vascular system and it allows the system to act more efficiently by allowing more blood flow and consequently more oxygen to the vital organs of the body including brain.

- Brain, being the highest oxygen consumer (20%) of the total oxygen requirement of the human body, regulates the body more efficiently.
- The improved blood circulation to brain including microcirculation in smaller capillaries increases memory and metabolic efficiency including neurotransmitters regulation.

- Ginkgo biloba is useful for relaxing coronary arteries constricted by cholesterol.

- Ginkgo biloba is also useful for relieving tension and anxiety.

- Ginkgo biloba is also beneficial to elevate mood and restore energy.

- Ginkgo biloba controls platelet activity factor (PAF). Excessive platelet factor (PAF) in the body may cause physical stress, brain disorder, and skin problem including psoriasis, cardiovascular disease and other hearing disorders.

- Ginkgo biloba is beneficial for treating vertigo and tinnitus.

- Ginkgo biloba acts as an antioxidant and inhibits free radical formed in the body. Antioxidant plays a vital role for protecting cardiovascular and central nervous system (CNS). The combined effect of improved circulatory system and antioxidant improves blood flow to retina and controls retinal deterioration causing an overall improvement in visual activity.

- Some of the clinical trials indicate that ginkgo biloba is beneficial for treating Alzheimer's disease.

- Ginkgo biloba is also used as supportive herbal medicine for treating infertility disorder in males.

Precaution:

Although it is a herbal medicine with enormous benefits, it should not be combined with certain antidepressants such as MAO (mono amine oxidase). Persons taking medicine for blood clotting disorders should avoid taking ginkgo biloba, as the medicine will increase the effect of prescribed medicine.
If you are pregnant or plan to become pregnant, you should not take ginkgo biloba.

Side Effects:

The possible side effects of the medicine include

- Ginkgo biloba may cause some gastrointestinal disorders.

- Ginkgo biloba increases the risk of bleeding and if you have or had any blood clotting disorder, you should not take ginkgo biloba.

- The other common side effects of ginkgo biloba may include nausea, diarrhea, vomiting, dizziness, headache and restlessness.

If you observe any of the side effect as mentioned above or any other side effect, you should stop taking ginkgo biloba and consult your doctor.

Bitter Melon - Medicinal Properties

Bitter Melon is reported to help in the treatment of diabetes and psoriasis. It has also been reported that Bitter Melon may help in the treatment of HIV. Bitter Melon is the English name of Momordica charantia. Bitter Melon is also known by the names Karela and Balsam Pear. Bitter Melon grows in tropical areas, including parts of East Africa, Asia, the Caribbean, and South America, where it is used as a food as well as a medicine.

It is a green cucumber shaped fruit with gourd-like bumps all over it. It looks like an ugly, light green cucumber. The fruit should be firm, like a cucumber. And it tastes very bitter. Although the seeds, leaves, and vines of Bitter Melon have all been used, the fruit is the safest and most prevalent part of the plant used medicinally. The leaves and fruit have both been used occasionally to make teas and beer, or to season soups in the Western world.

Bitter Melon was traditionally used for a dazzling array of conditions by people in tropical regions. Numerous infections, cancer, leukemia, and diabetes are among the most common conditions it was believed to improve.

Bitter Melon is reported to help in the treatment of diabetes and psoriasis. It has also been thought that Bitter Melon may help in the treatment of HIV, but the evidence thus far is too weak to even consider.

The ripe fruit of Bitter Melon has been suggested to exhibit some remarkable anti-cancer effects, but there is absolutely no evidence that it can treat cancer. However, preliminary studies do appear to confirm that Bitter Melon may improve blood sugar control in people with adult-onset (type 2) diabetes.

The blood lowering action of the fresh juice of the unripe Bitter Melon has been confirmed in scientific studies in animals and humans. At least three different groups of constituents in Bitter Melon have been reported to have hypoglycemic (blood sugar lowering) or other actions of potential benefit in diabetes mellitus.

These include a mixture of steroidal saponins known as charantin, insulin-like peptides, and alkaloids.
 It is still unclear which of these is most effective or if all three work together. Nonetheless, Bitter Melon preparations have been shown to significantly improve glucose tolerance without increasing blood insulin levels, and to improve fasting blood glucose levels.

Chakra Balancing

Chakra reconciliation is founded on the ancient Amerind impression in a series of 7 chakras, or vigor centers. Chakra is the Sanskrit word for wheel. These vigour centers ar believed to be placed at particular points between the pedestal of the spinal column and the circus tent of the skull. Some esoteric systems include additional chakras, said to extend beyond the tangible consistency into the human auric field.

Each chakra is believed to relate to particular organs of the consistence, ailments, colors, elements, and emotions. However, different systems or sources that use the idea of chakras whitethorn disagree about the details.

The conception of chakras plays a key role in two ancient Amerindian language healing systems (ayurvedic medicine and yoga) that popular today. In recent decades, however, many modern therapies (like polarity therapy, therapeutic touch, process acupressure, core energetics, and semblance therapy) rich person besides incorporated the idea of chakras into their own visions of healing.

Various approaches English hawthorn be used to "balance" the chakras. Chakra is believed to promote wellness by maximizing the stream of vim in the organic structure, much as a tune-up enables a car to operate on at peak efficiency. Chakras part of the ancient feeling arrangement connected with yoga.

These traditions were handed down orally for thousands of years before being codified by Patanjali in his Yoga Sutras, several centuries before Christ. The ancient healing science of Ayurveda is on a collection of scriptures known as vedas (a Sanskrit word meaning knowledge or wisdom). Ayurveda literally means "life knowledge."

It remained the predominant form of care in India until the British colonial government tried to suppress it during the nineteenth century. Over the last half-century, however, a modernized form of has gained considerable popularity in India.

More recently, traditional has been popularized in the West by such high-profile advocates as Deepak Chopra. Balancing the chakras is believed to promote general and well-being by ensuring the free flowing of life push (too known as prana or qi) throughout the physical structure. It is believed that blockages in the current of this vital get-up-and-go will eventually result in mental, emotional, and/or touchable illness.

By removing such blockages and Department of Energy menstruation, practitioners said to enable dead body, mind, and spirit to function optimally. Some alternative practitioners, such as medical intuitive, say they can "read" a patient's chakras to detect imbalances and diagnose problems.

This is likewise sometimes done using a pendulum. Just as the various forms of yoga attempt to mediate between the forcible and Negro spiritual realms, so the chakras believed to manoeuver as Energy Department transformers. They often shown as circles, spaced at intervals along the vertebral column, or sometimes as funnels of Energy.

Specific chants or sounds with the different chakras used in some yogic meditation practices as tools for healing and apparitional evolution. Each of the VII chakras is said to wealthy person physiological and metaphysical functions that relate to both the nature of the blockages and to the active problems they produce.

Chinese Food Therapy

In your quest to find more natural healing methods and natural supplements to good health, you're well advised to consider the ancient healing methods of the Chinese.

Chinese food therapy, also known as Chinese nutrition therapy, dates back to as early as 2000 BC, though proper documentation about its uses was found around 500 BC. In essence, Chinese food therapy involves the use of certain foods to aid in the healing of certain body ailments or assists in keeping healthy other bodily functions.

Followers of food therapy believe in the concept of yin and yang in food; the yin foods are believed to lower the body's metabolism, or decrease the body's heat, while the yang foods are said to increase the body's heat or increase metabolism.

The Chinese believe in four food groups, which are grains, vegetables, fruits and meats. There is no classification for dairy products, which are considered unsuitable for humans. The Chinese believe a balanced diet will consist of the following food combinations on a daily basis: 40 percent grains, 30 to 40 percent vegetables, 10 to 15 percent meats and the rest of the foods should be nuts and fruits.

In Chinese food therapy, foods are then further classified by taste. The tastes are defined as pungent, salty, bitter, sweet and sour. Each taste is believed to have a direct effect on a body organ; when consumed in moderation it benefits the organ, but if over consumed, can cause detrimental effect to the organ.

It's fair to say the Chinese and followers of Chinese food therapy truly believe you "are what you eat".

One simple example of Chinese food therapy is the remedy for a cough. The Cantonese cough remedy required apricot kernels, watercress and dried duck gizzards.

The ingredients are slow cooked for several hours, and a bit of pork can be added for flavor (though you can't add beef or chicken because both will nullify the healing effects of the watercress). The watercress removes the excessive amount of yang in the body, while the duck gizzards are added to balance the yin yang of the recipe. The apricots target the lungs.

Take the time to learn from Chinese healing wisdom - you may just be surprised how it benefits your health.

Natural Medicine Vs Chemically Produced Medicine

Natural alternative medicines now are receiving a lot of build-up and hype and regular medicine are now receiving a lot of flak as well. This is brought upon by the many cases of side effects that might as well do more harm than good. People are rediscovering the goodness of what is natural and chemical-free.

Knowing that these natural alternative medicines were used for centuries upon centuries already makes them more reliable than prescription drugs for many people. Also, the fact that the list of benefits hugely overrates the harm, which rarely happens, gives a great reason to give it at least a try. Nothing is lost and everything is to be gained.

But who's to say which is really best for us, regular or natural alternative medicines? Many or most of us generally rely on doctors to tell us what to do and which medicine to use. Well, this is the best choice, but seeking a second opinion may also be very recommendable especially if your doctor couldn't or is having a hard time curing you.

There are a lot of differences between regular prescription medicines and natural alternative medicines. But the main factor that drives people away is not only their price difference but also their effectiveness and the barrage of side effects. Natural alternative medicine has been proven and tested with age and time already.

Aside from the herbs and spices and teas, natural alternative medicine can be coupled with massages, mental exercises such as meditation, aromatherapies and so much more. Many regular medicines have come and gone but natural alternative medicines have lived on. The main reason for this is because we know that they work.

Cleansing Liver - Herbal Teas

When spring comes it is time for a liver cleanse. This is a good time to rejuvenate the liver for the coming year of work. One good way to cleanse the liver is to use herbal teas. They are easy to use and they provide a powerful punch to reawaken the liver.

Here is a herbal formulation for the liver provided by Brigitte Mars (herbalist in Colorado) called "Puri-Tea" which consist of:

- Peppermint, red clover, fennel, licorice
- cleavers, dandelion, oregon grape root, burdock root
- butternut bark, chickweed, parsley root, nettles.

Another liver herbal tea is:

- Fennel Seed (1 part), Fenugreek (1 part)
- Flax Seed (1 part), Licorice Root (1/4 part)
- Burdock (1/4 part), Peppermint (1 part).

Here's another herbal combination that is good for detoxifying and cleansing the liver:

- Yellow Dock root, Dandelion root, Licorice root
- Red sage, Sarsaparilla, Hyssop
- Pau de Arco, Milk Thistle Seed, Parsley leaf.

Here's something else you can do for you liver. Buy an extract of Milk Thistle Seed. Then when you make the liver tea's list here, add 2-3 full droppers of the Milk Thistle Seed extract to the tea.
Here are the effects of some of the herbs listed above.

- fennel seed - white cell formation, acid/alkaline balancing

- peppermint - body cleanser and toner
- red clover - blood purifier
- licorice - adrenal stimulation
- cleavers - anti-infection
- dandelion - cleansing and strengthening
- oregon grape root - cleansing, building
- burdock root - purifying
- nettles - rich in minerals
- chickweed -
- fenugreek - helps to eliminate toxins and mucus
- yellow dock root - cleansing, white cell formation
- pau de arco - cleansing, white cell formation
- milk thistle seed - cleansing, building

You can make these teas yourself or look for a readymade one at a health food store. What I do is buy a 1/2 or 1 oz of each herb. Then I mix one full tablespoon of each herb into a mason jar. Shake it up and its ready to go. Preparing the tea

Boil 1 1/4 cup of distilled water in a glass container. Add 1 heaping tablespoon of herbal mixture. Let tea sit for 10-15 minutes. Strain and drink when it cools down a little.
Drink one cup of tea before breakfast and one before dinner for about 1-2 months.

Colon Cleanse

Colon cleansing has been in the news among health enthusiasts for some time because it can offer relief for a variety of symptoms. The reason for this is that the intestinal tract commonly becomes impacted with fecal matter, which in turn releases toxins (poisons) into the bloodstream. While constipation is obviously a primary symptom of this state of affairs, other symptoms can be traced to the released poisons.

Some of the symptoms that have also been connected to an impacted bowel include headaches, fatigue, depression, and allergy symptoms. Weight gain and an inability to lose it are also associated with an impacted bowel. In addition, people report nervous symptoms like irritability and "walking around in a fog." Feeling "bloated" with gas is another common symptom, and some people even report problems with their skin.

The traditional methods have included increasing the fiber in the diet while taking laxative herbs, such as Cascara Sagrada or Senna. These laxatives are harsh to the body and can create a dependency not unlike an addiction. Fiber for constipation usually is made up of psyllium seed husks.

This natural plant derivative absorbs water in the bowel and becomes mucilaginous. This creates a bulk that is helpful for removing matter from the colon, but it is not a complete cleanse.

A lesser known method, oxygen based colon cleansing, is also taken orally, but does not work on the same principle as the fiber and herb method. This method uses an "oxidation reduction" type of chemical reaction to melt away the material in the bowel. Because the reaction gives off oxygen, which is then absorbed into the body, it is healthful and energizing.

Another option in traditional treatment of an impacted bowel is to take enemas or colonic irrigation. These methods force water, herbal teas, or other medications up into the digestive tract through a tube inserted into the rectal cavity.

Colonic irrigation goes farther up into the intestines than does an enema. It should be done by a licensed professional. Obviously, this is an unpleasant matter at best, but can be helpful when used in conjunction with oxygen based colon cleansing.

The best option for dealing with constipation and the other symptoms of an impacted bowel is to use an oxygen based colon cleansing product. The best of these will contain the mineral germanium in an organic form. This mineral, which is sometimes called Ge-132, is found in some of the most healthful food and herbs around, including garlic, comfrey, watercress, ginseng, and certain edible fungi (mushrooms.)

Having germanium in your colon cleanse can help lower blood pressure, improve artery health, and lower cholesterol. It is thought to be anti-carcinogenic, or an agent to prevent various cancers.

It helps the colon cleanse to create even more oxygen, which brings life and health to the internal organs. Germanium is also helpful for reducing the growth of the yeast, Candida albicans, in the body. Candida has been associated with symptoms such as fatigue, itching, headaches, and a host of others.

Comfrey - For The Mother To Be

Comfrey
(Symphytum Officinale)

Medicinal Parts: Rootstock, leaves

Description: Comfrey is a perennial plant common in moist meadows and other moist places in the U.S. and Europe.

Properties: anodyne, astringent, demulcent, emollient, expectorant, hemostatic, refrigerant, vulnerary.

Comfrey is truly one of nature's miracle cures. The root produces a high amount of a gummy material called mucilage, and the root and leaf are both high in allantoin, a substance that helps with cell proliferation. Comfrey is excellent for reducing the swelling around a fracture, thereby allowing the union to take place with greater facility.

And according to herbalist John Gerard, "A salve concocted from the fresh herb will certainly tend to promote the healing of bruised and broken parts."

My midwife first introduced me to Comfrey after the birth of my first child. To put it mildly, it was not an easy delivery. All of those little joys after childbirth were making me very uncomfortable. You know the tearing, bruising, stitches, etc. The midwife instructed me to steep Comfrey leaves in hot water and add it to my sitz bath. The results were phenomenal. It relieved the discomfort almost instantaneously.

Today, any time I attend a baby shower, I make up a gift basket stocked with comfrey. I wrap a generous handful of comfrey leaves in

cheesecloth, then tie it closed with a ribbon. The packets can then be tossed directly into a pot of water to steep.

Recipients always think I'm a bit odd at first, but usually I receive a heartfelt thank you note a couple of weeks after the baby is born. This is one gift any mother-to-be will appreciate.

Cure for the Common Cold

A co-worker of mine once had a troublesome cold a while back for weeks on end and because I had to add to my workload by splitting his share up with the rest in the office, I told him of a method to use as a cure for the common cold used by the Indians and some West Africans. (Okay, I'm not that insensitive-I told him this because I cared!)

This method is known in Sanskrit (the Indian Language) as Neti or "Nasal Irrigation).

It is the cleaning of the nasal portion of the respiratory system whose function is to allow air to come in contact with the circulating blood so exchange of the gases can happen.

If this sounds a little bit complex if you need a cure for your cold and are not trying to read all these facts, just believe this works as a cure for the common cold the way nothing else can. (well besides a fast...)

Neti (nasal irrigation) is unmatched in its ability to
-Clear the nostrils for freer breathing.
-Reduce excess mucus.
-Moisten the nasal canal; strengthen the eyes, because there is stimulation of the blood vessels of the nose and eyes via nasal irrigation.

Cure for the Common cold: Using Nasal irrigation (neti)

1. Using un-iodized TABLE SALT, add a level teaspoon of salt to 24 oz warm water.
2. Wash your neti pot (which is available in most health food stores).
3. Re- rinse internally and externally with drinking water.
4. Fill the pot (which holds about 8 oz) with the saline solution

5. Now tilt your head so your right nostril is uppermost over a sink or large basin
6. Pour the solution into the nostril and ensure to keep the mouth open to breathe.
7. After it all comes out, remain motionless for 30 seconds or so then blow the nose
Thoroughly and rinse out the mouth with drinking water.

Repeat steps 1-7 on the right nostril pouring through the left this time.

You can bend forward to ensure it all drips out or preferably perform 10-15 rounds of bellows breath (a breathing exercise that entails forcefully pulling the belly back towards the spine which pushes the stagnant air out of the lungs) to get all the solution out.

I found it pleasant and soothing after practicing it only once. Besides aiding as a cure for the common cold, it also ensures that blocked nasal passages as a result of irritants and pollutants are well loosened.

Furthermore it is said to have a marked cleansing effect on the sinuses and mind and helps to clean the anterior regions of the upper palate housing the olfactory organs. It even helps to cleanse to some degree the inner workings of the ear. Children using this product should be supervised by an able adult.
Cure for the Common Cold: Dietetic Suggestions

Moreover, to target the root cause of the common cold, now will be a good time to try one kind of a fast which could be
1.   The use of Fresh Fruit juices.
2.   The Broth of succulent and tasty steamed vegetables such as celery, cabbage etc
3.   A mono-diet of a seasonal juicy fruit.

If like most people, you just cannot fast, we'll see to it that you abstain from all types of Animal Products, Breads, Grains and beans during this time. These substances have been known to either cause or aggravate the common cold along with other diseases and conditions including but not limited to the flu, asthma and diabetes.

This fact is based on research performed the renowned French Hygienist, Albert Mosseri. A good replacement for the less beneficial items listed above will be fresh fruits, roots and leafy vegetables for fuel.

So don't be fooled into spending your money on drugs and nasal sprays as a cure for the common cold, it, like any other disease, can be alleviated by common-sense drugless healing alternatives, if only you know how.

With the steps above, you, like my co-worker, now know exactly how to cure you cold naturally for long-term success.

Detox Diet

Juice fasting is gaining popularity as a great way to detoxify. Many people are interested in getting toxins out of their system so they can live a healthier life. When toxins accumulate in the body, they feel sluggish and also have a poor immune system. Juice fasting, as a cleansing method, can help to people to achieve better health and more energy. It is quite easy to do as fruits are readily obtainable and all that is required additionally is a juicer.

For a beginner to juice fasting, it is important to start out slow and to try it out for one day. By juice fasting, you are limiting your intake to juices only. Fruit juice is high in sugar, so if you are a diabetic or otherwise in need of monitoring your sugar intake you should be cautious of trying a juice fast with fruit juices.

Anyone just starting out with fasting should always speak with their doctor first. Also, do not juice fast for prolonged periods like more than 3 days, not unless your doctor agrees that it is safe for you to do so.

The following are sample recipes that can help give you an idea of combinations of fruits and vegetables to use together:

Recipe 1: Vegetable Juice Combo
2 Swiss chard leaves
1/2 beetroot
2 or 3 sprigs of watercress
3 carrots
1 celery stalk
Wash with filtered or distilled water, cut and put in juicer.

Recipe 2: Carrot-Apple Juice
2-3 Green Apples
1 carrot
Fresh basil leaves
Wash with filtered or distilled water, cut and put in juicer.

Recipe 3: Carrot-Vegetable Juice
A handful of dandelion leaves
1 kale leaf
4 carrots
Fresh mint, basil or coriander leaves
Wash with filtered or distilled water, cut and put in juicer.

Recipe 4: Peach Juice
2 or 3 peaches
Wash with filtered or distilled water, cut and put in juicer.

There are many different types of juice fasts. Some diets call for fruit juices while others used less sugary vegetable juices. You can always come up with your own unique combination of fruit and vegetable juice diet recipes.

Eat Bran to Eliminate Constipation

One reason many people are constipated is they don't eat a lot of fiber. Most people only eat about 8 mg of fiber per day. To have good health and have good elimination, you need around 30- 35 mg of fiber.

Eating bran is one of the quickest and best ways to increase your fiber. It will increase the weight and size of your stools more than the fiber contained in fruits or vegetables. Bran is the outer husk of the grain - wheat, corn, rice, and oat - which is indigestible.

It does not irritate the lining of the stomach, small intestine or your colon. It is not a laxative but promotes the movement fecal matter through your colon in a natural way. Unlike drugstore laxatives or other natural strong laxatives, bran does not quickly purge out all the contents in your colon.

Use one or two heaping tablespoon of bran in your morning cereal, in your baking, and in your smoothies.

Health Alert: When using bran, make sure you drink plenty of water during the day to keep your stools soft.

Here are some other ways to use bran. You can add them to,

"   baked breads, muffins and other baked goods
"   breaded mixes
"   hamburger meat
"   juices
"   pancake or waffle mix
"   salads
"   scramble eggs
"   soups
"   soups

"   stuffing
"   vegetarian burger mix
"   yogurt

When you put bran in juices or anything that is all liquid just eat it with a spoon.

How much bran should you take for good bowel regularity? Each person is different. You need to experiment. Start with two teaspoon each day and work towards 10 teaspoons a day or until you have bowel movements without effort or straining.

There are four basic bran products - wheat, corn, oat, and rice. They all provide a solid source of fiber in varying amounts. Make sure the bran you use is 100% unprocessed bran.

Use bran for a few weeks to get your bowel movements back to normal. Eating bran should get your bowels moving in a few days or less.

Once your bowels are back to normal, back off from using a lot of bran and depend more on fiber from eating more fruits, vegetables, nuts, and seeds.

There are many new products, which use bran added to other nutrients or powders. Although these can be useful, use them for a limit time.

Eczema and Psoriasis

The purpose of this article is to tell the world what I have learned from my own personal experience about an inexpensive and effective treatment for eczema. Because psoriasis is a very similar affliction, there's a good chance that this treatment would be effective for psoriasis too.

Eczema is a skin irritation characterized by red, flaky skin that sometimes has cracks or tiny blisters. It's believed to be hereditary and if both parents have it, there is an 80% chance that their children will have it too.

Once upon a time, I had medical insurance coverage and I was able to afford any medication my doctor prescribed. I used to have a slew of little bottles and creams that were somewhat effective in relieving the itching, but nothing I ever tried had any effect whatsoever in terms of reducing the severity or frequency of eczema attacks.

Topical applications of cortisone cream have a limited effect in terms of relieving the itching, but cortisone just suppresses eczema and can actually cause it to spread. There's a theory that eczema can be brought on by stress, and I believe that may be true.

After experiencing a yearlong constant virulent attack during 2004 through 2005 when I was under severe stress, I decided to seek medical help in order to find out whether anything new had been discovered regarding eczema treatment.

The only treatment I didn't already know about involves exposure to ultraviolet light radiation which is very expensive. For many years there have been medications that are taken internally, but all of them require regular blood testing for possible liver damage. For me, this is out of the question because any medication that is capable of causing liver damage comes under the category of unacceptable.

One day I was returning from a doctor visit when I passed a health food store, and I had some time to spend so I went in.

The woman behind the counter turned out to be a certified nutritionist so I asked her whether she knew anything about eczema treatment that the doctors don't know about.

She said "Yes, I do." I said "Really. Tell me." She brought out a small bottle of liquid zinc and told me that some of her customers had reported success with topical applications on their eczema sores. So I bought a bottle. I figured "What have I got to lose? Nothing. Twenty bucks, maybe." To my surprise, it relieved the itching and seemed to have some limited effect in reducing the inflammations.

The health food store lady had told me that zinc is a healer so I started thinking about it. I remembered that Desitin is a very effective and well known treatment for baby rash and that the active ingredient is zinc oxide. I thought "If liquid zinc is effective topically, how much more effective could it be if I take it internally?" Being inherently cheap, I was a bit bothered by the idea of buying another small bottle of liquid zinc and I knew that zinc tablets are inexpensive.

And that certainly appealed to my wallet. I discussed my idea with the nutritionist who agreed that it could work. So I began with the 75 mg. daily dose that the woman recommended and gradually worked my way upwards until I reached 200 mg. a day.

Eczema makes me so angry that I often curse "the eczema Nazis" each time the first blister occurs with the unmistakable itch that feels like it originates in my bones. I say to myself, "Damnation, I'm under attack again!" Now I say "Come on zinc, be John Wayne and kill every last one of those eczema Nazis!" Eight months after I began my inexpensive experiment with zinc taken internally, I can report real progress.

Where previously one tiny eczema blister always signaled a serious outbreak, now it stops without spreading any further and heals very quickly. The indicative first blister is not necessarily accompanied by itching either. To me, this is very significant because it constitutes a completely new pattern that has never before manifested in my entire life.

If you want to try taking zinc internally, I'd recommend "chelated" zinc because zinc is a mineral and minerals are not easily absorbed into the bloodstream. Back in the early 1980's, the health food industry discovered that if minerals are chemically linked to something the body can easily absorb, they are far more effective.

The chemists who invent these things decided to use amino acids which are natural proteins, and proteins are easily absorbable. The process of chemically linking a mineral to an amino acid is called chelation.

Effexor XR - a Potent Inhibitor

Effexor XR is a potent inhibitor of the reuptake of serotonin and norepinephrine-two neurotransmitters thought to play important roles in the pathophysiology of depression. Correcting the imbalance of these two chemicals may help relieve symptoms of depression.

How Taken

Effexor XR comes as a capsule to take by mouth. It is usually taken once a day and should be taken with food. Each capsule should be swallowed whole with fluid and not divided, crushed, chewed, or placed in water, or it may be administered by carefully opening the capsule and sprinkling the entire contents on a spoonful of applesauce.

This drug/food mixture should be swallowed immediately without chewing and followed with a glass of water to ensure complete swallowing of the pellets.

Warnings/Precautions

Before starting Effexor XR, tell your doctor about any medicines you're taking, including over-the-counter drugs and herbal supplements. If you take MAOIs you should not take Effexor XR. If you are taking antidepressants you should be watched closely for signs that your condition is getting worse or that you are becoming suicidal, especially when you first start therapy, or when your dose is increased or decreased.

You should also be watched for becoming agitated, irritable, hostile, impulsive, or restless. Such symptoms should be reported to your doctor right away. Effexor XR may raise blood pressure in some patients, so blood pressure should be monitored regularly.

When you suddenly stop using or quickly lower your daily dose of Effexor XR, discontinuation symptoms may occur. Talk to your doctor before discontinuing or reducing your dose of Effexor XR. Pregnant or nursing women shouldn't take any antidepressant without consulting their doctor. Until you see how Effexor XR affects you, be careful doing such activities as driving a car or operating machinery. Avoid drinking alcohol while taking Effexor XR.

Missed Dose

Take the missed dose as soon as you remember. However, if it is almost time for the next dose, skip the missed dose and take only the next one as directed. Do not take a double dose of this medication.

Possible Side Effects

If you experience any of the following serious side effects, stop taking Effexor XR and contact your doctor immediately or seek emergency medical treatment: an allergic reaction (difficulty breathing; closing of the throat; swelling of the lips, tongue, or face; or hives); seizures; or an irregular heartbeat or severely high blood pressure (blurred vision, headache).

Other, less serious side effects may be more likely to occur. Continue to take Effexor XR and talk to your doctor if you experience nausea, vomiting, upset stomach, abdominal pain, or loss of appetite or weight; dry mouth; drowsiness or dizziness; mild tremor, anxiety, or agitation; insomnia; abnormal dreams; sexual problems such as impotence, abnormal ejaculation, difficulty reaching orgasm, or decreased libido; sweating; yawning; or increase in blood cholesterol levels (detected by blood tests).

Side effects other than those listed here may also occur. Talk to your doctor about any side effect that seems unusual or that is especially bothersome.

Managing Pain

Perhaps the hardest part of having arthritis or a related condition is the pain that usually accompanies it. Managing and understanding that pain, and the impact it has on one's life, is a big issue with most arthritis sufferers. The first step in managing arthritis pain is knowing which type of arthritis or condition you have, because that will help determine your treatment. Before learning different management techniques, however, it's important to understand some concepts about pain.

No. 1: Not All Pain is Alike

Just as there are different types of arthritis, there are also different types of pain. Even your own pain may vary from day to day.

No. 2: The Purpose of Pain

Pain is your body's way of telling you that something is wrong, or that you need to act. If you touch a hot stove, pain signals from your brain tell you to pull your hand away. This type of pain helps protect you. Chronic, long-lasting pain, like the kind that accompanies arthritis, is different. While it tells you that something is wrong, it often isn't as easy to relieve.

No. 3: Causes of Pain

Arthritis pain is caused by several factors, such as (1) Inflammation, the process that causes the redness and swelling in your joints; (2) Damage to joint tissues, which results from the disease process or from stress, injury or pressure on the joints; (3) Fatigue resulting from the disease process, which can make pain worse and more difficult to bear; and (4) Depression or stress, which results from limited movement or no longer doing activities you enjoy.

No. 4: Pain Factors

Things such as stress, anxiety, depression or simply "overdoing it" can make pain worse. This often leads to a decrease in physical activity, causing further anxiety and depression, resulting in a downward spiral of ever-increasing pain.

No. 5: Different Reactions to Pain

People react differently to pain. Mentally, you can get caught in a cycle of pain, stress and depression, often resulting from the inability to perform certain functions, which makes managing pain and arthritis seem more difficult. Physically, pain increases the sensitivity of your nervous system and the severity of your arthritis.

Emotional and social factors include your fears and anxieties about pain, previous experiences with pain, energy level, attitude about your condition and the way people around you react to pain.

No. 6: Managing Your Pain

Arthritis may limit some of the things you can do, but it doesn't have to control your life. One way to reduce your pain is to build your life around wellness, not pain or sickness. This means taking positive action. Your mind plays an important role in how you feel pain and respond to illness.

Many people with arthritis have found that by learning and practicing pain management skills, they can reduce their pain. Thinking of pain as a signal to take positive action rather than an ordeal you have to endure can help you learn to manage your pain. You can counteract the downward spiral of pain by practicing relaxation techniques, regular massage, hot and cold packs, moderate exercise, and keeping a positive mental outlook. And humor always has a cathartic effect.

No. 7: Don't focus on pain.

The amount of time you spend thinking about pain has a lot to do with how much discomfort you feel. People who dwell on their pain usually say their pain is worse than those who don't dwell on it. One way to take your mind off pain is to distract yourself from pain. Focus on something outside your body, perhaps a hobby or something of personal interest, to take your mind off your discomfort.

No. 8: Think positively.

What we say to ourselves often determines what we do and how we look at life. A positive outlook will get you feeling better about yourself, and help to take your mind off your pain. Conversely, a negative outlook sends messages to yourself that often lead to increased pain, or at least the feeling that the pain is worse. So, "in with the good, and out with the bad."

Reinforce your positive attitude by rewarding yourself each time you think about or do something positive. Take more time for yourself. Talk to your doctor about additional ways to manage pain.

Acupunture

Emotional Freedom Techniques (EFT) is a healing tool based on the theory that our emotions and physical symptoms are linked to the underlying energy system of the body. That energy system is the acupuncture meridian system known to the Chinese for thousands of years.

EFT was developed by Stanford Engineer Gary Craig, who discovered the basic theory in 1991 and continues to this day to develop and improve on EFT applications.

The underpinning theory of EFT is simple, yet sheds a whole new light on our emotional experiences and how we interpret them.

Gary Craig's EFT discovery statement asserts that: "The cause of all negative emotions is a disruption in the body's energy system." He believes that "our unresolved negative emotions are major contributors to most physical pains and diseases."

How Does EFT Work?

Chinese Medicine and the ancient Indian Science of Ayurveda both support the concept that our emotional experiences, in particular resentments, hurts and anger, contribute significantly to the development of disease in the human body.

While the EFT theory that all negative emotions are caused by a disruption in the energy system of the body may sound odd at first, the idea is far from new. In fact, it's 5,000 years old and was more recently enforced by Albert Einstein who taught that everything is made of energy.

The reason EFT works so well is purely because it embraces the secrets of Eastern healing traditions that have been overlooked by the west.

Acupuncture is finally attracting interest, and research has been conducted to try and figure out how and why it works. Yet that research will always seek to put acupuncture in a box that makes sense to what conforms in the West. The impressive results of acupuncture have been called a placebo effect, when, in truth, they are due to an ancient understanding of meridian energy circuitry which runs throughout all living creatures.

EFT & Acupuncture

In acupuncture, points are carefully selected by practitioners trained to read the maps of the meridian system. EFT is based on a select few of these potent points known to excel in giving emotional and physical relief to anyone who simply learns where they are and how to use them. EFT doesn't require expert knowledge, or the use of needles, the points are simply stimulated by tapping on them with the fingertips.

We need only look to the fact that in China hundreds of people every day undergo heart surgery using nothing but acupuncture for anesthesia, to realize that anything based on the solid healing foundation that acupuncture has to offer is worth exploring further.

Gary Craig developed EFT as an incredibly user friendly access point to the benefits of acupuncture and the healing potential latent within us all to deal with our physical and emotional pain. EFT's track record for relieving negative emotions, anxiety and trauma has earned it the descriptive title of "acupuncture for the emotions, but without the needles."

The EFT Challenge

There's an old saying that we should judge a tree by its fruits. The fruits of EFT can be quickly and easily tasted by learning the basics and setting EFT to work on dissolving any negative emotion. EFT takes just 5 minutes to learn, and then you can put it to the test of your own direct experience.

Finding A Natural Remedy Isn't Difficult

Finding a natural remedy to sickness or an ailment isn't hard. A quick visit to a health food store to speak with a clerk who is well versed in what herbs are natural remedies for what ailment can provide a wealth of knowledge. Also a quick surfing tour of the internet using natural remedy as a keyword for the search can provide a great deal of knowledge.

When looking for a natural remedy use common sense and add a grain of salt to what you may be told. Some people take it to an extreme and think there is a natural remedy for everything. Not true, but if you use common sense you'll probably find a natural remedy for most ailments.

After all, for many hundreds of years there was no such thing as a pharmaceutical industry, and using a natural remedy to cure an illness was the only way an illness could be cured.

The world of the natural remedy is varied and multi faceted. A few examples however are very common and should be known by everyone. For instance, zinc is a great natural remedy for colds. Cranberries are a natural remedy for urinary track infections, especially common for women.

Aloe Vera juice applied to cuts and abrasions is a natural remedy that does wonders for healing. Garlic is a natural remedy for heart disease and an immune system strengthening agent. Seeds from the common pumpkin are a natural remedy to rid the body of parasites.

Apple cider vinegar is a multifunctional natural remedy for many diseases, and an overall cleanser of the system. St. John's Wort is a natural remedy for depression symptoms. Oranges, lemons, limes, grapefruit, and other citrus fruits are full of vitamins and a great natural remedy for the common cold, as is chicken soup. White vinegar is a natural remedy for toe fungus when the feet are soaked in it.

Cinnamon is a natural remedy for high blood pressure and much safer than pharmacological solutions. Grape seed is an ancient natural remedy for prostate problems, common in middle aged and older men. Finding a natural remedy is tea is easy. Green tea boosts the immune system, ginger tea aids digestion, and most teas in general help keep the system flushed out and pure. With this entire in mind, it is easy to see that a natural remedy is usually an option for almost any minor health problem.

Foot Massage

Foot massage or foot reflexology has a Chinese origin. It dates back to more than 3,000 years ago and is used in the prevention and cure of many health ailments.

Some in fact say, foot massage dates back to ancient Egyptian times due to archaeological findings in cave drawings in Egypt.

The principle of foot massage rests in the premise that the meridian network connects all tissues, organs and cells in our body. Each organ in the body is connected to a specific reflex point on the foot through the intermediary of 300 nerves. A trained foot reflexologist can put pressure on different meridians or energy lines on the sole and side of the feet to determine the cause of illness.

By using pressure to these the reflex points, the foot massage is good for stimulating the activity internal organs, and to improve blood and lymph circulation. Thus, the top to bottom well being of a person can be made through the foot.

The principles of foot massage are not in congruence with western allopathic medicine. Western medicine merely sees the foot as a body part comprising of bones, ligaments and joints.

However, foot massage is fast gaining much popularity and acceptance as an alternative health treatment. Fans of foot massage believe it can cure not only colds and minor ailments, but more serious ailments as well. These ailments include liver dysfunction, constipation problems, chronic headaches, skin allergies, etc.

Like most Oriental medical techniques, foot reflexology is a "holistic" treatment. It concentrates on treating the whole person rather than just the symptoms of one particular ailment.

While Western medicine promises speedy recovery of all unpleasant symptoms, foot massage therapy can be slow and gradual. A series of visits is necessary to strengthen the body and to bring the body back to balance.

A session of foot reflexology in San Francisco, can set you back as much as $40-100. Thus, foot massages over a period of time, can add up in terms of costs.

However, for practitioners and believers of foot massage, the cost for good health is well worth it. The alternative would have been money spent in clinics and western hospitals for prescription drugs and perhaps, invasive surgery.

Creative Steps To Healing

Ever have the feeling that disease was controlling your life? Perhaps it's not even a chronic illness. Do you harbor anger? Resentment? Frustration?

Maybe it's just me and I'm talking to myself, but I've let these entire rule my life at some point. Therefore, in this short article, I thought we'd take a look at "Four Creative Steps To Healing." From it, I hope you'll gain insight into yourself, your behaviors and perhaps the way you deposit or withdraw from your own health currency.

Step One: Understand Your Energy

We've all heard about the aura that surrounds the body, but what could this possibly have to do with our health?

Translation: These cycles or waves of energy that surround our body are a function of our thoughts. Thoughts are energy waves then, that affect our health in a positive or negative way. Let's look a little closer to see why this happens:

The contributors to this energy surrounding the body are the 7 major "chakras" (chakra in Sanskrit means "wheel or vortex").

It has been shown scientifically that each of these 7 wheels of energy corresponds to a particular endocrine gland in the body. Translation: In light of the adage, "you are what you eat" we could conclude with with some degree of certainty that "you are what you think."

Now that you've been (hopefully) examining your thoughts and translating all of your negative energy into positive. Would you agree that "healing is unattractive?" I needed some time to think about this: Why in the world would healing be unattractive?
Answer Our wounds give us power! And after careful contemplation, I've outlined three ways I have done this, myself.

Ask yourself: Are you leading with your wounds? You'll know if you done any of the following:

1. Used Wounds to Manipulate a Situation or a Person.

Let's say we find a situation unsavory, scary or inflaming a personal "hot button." Have you ever avoided a situation when you really needed to face head on? Or, how 'bout this one: "I just can't get into this relationship - I've been burned before!" Okay, maybe I am just speaking to myself here, but I admit, I've used my wounds (more times than I care to admit) to refrain from loving unconditionally.

2. Use Them to Attract Other Wounded Souls Who Want to Exchange in the "Wound" Game.

I've done this myself, too. In listening to another share their wounds, I've given up compassion for wound ante – "Ill see you and raise you one." Agreed, there is a difference between healing from a wound and "leading with a wound" but, in my humble opinion, I'd be willing to bet that we know the difference between being healthy and not.

For example, I know when I'm healthy when I can listen with empathy, void of getting out my toolbox to "fix" or laying out my wounds unsolicited.

3. Give Up Our Ability to Listen.

Dr. Bernie Siegel in his book "Peace, Love and Healing" basically says, listening is the work of angels. Many times listening is all we have in a situation when someone calls on us for help.

While listening attentively, my mind searched its experiences for a similar event. All this so I could say: "Oh that's terrible! Don't feel so bad though, because I've been through this thing that is so much worse!"

To reclaim my character, however, (and after I realized what was happening), I caught myself. In reality, all this person really needed was my ear to listen unconditionally.

Step Three: Learn To Forgive Yourself and Others

The final two steps are remedies which can help heal our anger, resentment and frustration. Step three then, is simply forgiveness. For to forgive in earnest then takes our energy out of its emotional investment in the past.

We give up the need to spend wasted energy making negative deposits into this account and, is the fastest way to bring our energy into real time. Translation: Trust me, you'll know authentic forgiveness when you experience it. The body literally "lets go" of the weight of the past.

Step Four: Love Yourself

The final creative step to healing? Loving yourself, of course! This is the most challenging concept, in my opinion. Why? To begin we must start where we are, and love and accept ourselves for who we are, today. How does this help our health? It's simple, when we realize that we are stunting our personal growth and health through negative self talk, we can then begin to love ourselves one piece at a time.

Here's how it's done (Author's note: beware, this practice may seem untraditional yet, if you'll consult Louise L. Hay's book: "You Can Heal Your Life" - you'll find that this is one of the remedies she used to heal herself from cancer):

Every day spend 15 minutes in the mirror sending love to you! Start small by finding one part of yourself where you can find perfection. Each day, or week, or months choose new parts of yourself to love. Before long, you'll find an image of perfection before your eyes. And you'll have purified your energy, to boot!

In closing, we could make all of these steps very simple, indeed. For there is only one step here that will make you healthy and happy. Remember: It's when we've learned to love ourselves that we can truly be healed.

Fruit Extracts – Prevent Aging of Skin

Are the growing wrinkles on your face giving you sleepless nights? Cosmetic market is flooded with innumerable types of lotions and creams that give assurance of reducing the wrinkles helping you look young. But, these cosmetic products contain harmful chemicals which may help you at present but can harm your skin in the future.

At this point of time a question may arise in your mind that – "Is there any other alternative or option which can help you, without leaving any adverse affect"? Yes, the answer is "fruit extracts" that can help you look younger and that too a natural way.

Fruit extracts are prepared from fruits with little or no outside ingredients. Fruits such as apple, banana, custard apple, guava, lime, mango alphonso, orange, papaya, pineapple, strawberry are commonly used for making fruit extracts products.

Use of fruits in cosmetic functions is mainly due to the presence of vitamins and alpha hydroxyl acids (AHA) such as glycolic, lactic, malic, citric and tartaric acids. Fruit extracts are known to have refreshing, purifying as well as soothing and hydrating properties. They are used for caring and grooming body, skin and hair.

Variety of fruit extracts are available in the market to suit perfectly to all skin types and hair texture. Deciding which fruit extract product to buy and from where must be bewildering you by now.

Let me firstly answer the former part of the question. To find which fruit extract to buy, you initially need to do a bit of research. Find what type is of skin texture do you have is it oily, dry or normal. If this task seems tough, you can seek for this information from professional advice from cosmetologist, who can guide you in a better manner that which fruit extract product will suit your skin type.

The next thing you need to do is to search through the market about all the available sellers or companies of the particular fruit extract that you are looking for. You can go out and can shop for them in the cosmetic shop but in case you don't want to get into all these hassles, you can look for online cosmetic sellers. Now a day's number of well known companies have open up their websites, so that a customer can look at all the products they offer at one place.

Go through the various websites, you can read the feature of each fruit extract and can find the suitable fruit extract product that suits your needs to the best and that too at a much lower price than that available in the open market.

Growth of the fruit extracts usage in other words organic food segment has bang upon the "natural cosmetics" industry by raising consumers' expectations. The positive image of fruits positive in food has now moved across to cosmetic products such as fruit extracts and many more. Get a new young look with fruit extracts and let other guess what your right age is.

Fruits and Juices for Relieving Hemorrhoids

Chili Peppers

It has been found that when you eat a lot of chili peppers that you can get a burning sensation in the rectum or anus. It is best to avoid eating too many peppers, especially if you have an advance case of hemorrhoids. Peppers are actually good for blood circulation and for healing ulcers. It is always the excess that creates problems in your body.

Here are some additional foods to avoid, which cause constipation.

• Coffee
• Alcohol
• Bad Fats
• Animal products
• Red meat

Foods you should be eating to help relieve hemorrhoids

A high fiber diet obtained from raw fruits and vegetables is what you need to eat for eliminating and for preventing constipation. When you don't have constipation, you won't have hemorrhoids.

The amount of fiber you should be eating is 25- 35 grams per day. Most people only eat about 8 – 12 grams per day.

If you have not been eating a lot of fiber, you need to add fiber slowly to your diet, especially if you add it by using bran. Increase your use of bran or other bran cereals over a couple of weeks.

If you add fiber to your diet with fruits and vegetables, you can add them freely without much problem. However, since your stomach will not be use to it, you may experience more gas for a week or two. You can compensate for this by taking digestive enzymes to help you digest the extra produce.

The following list of juices and fruits are good for helping cure or relieve hemorrhoids.

Juices

Juices are good for hemorrhoids but especially dark berry juices mixed with equal parts of apple juice. The dark berry juices to use are, cherries, blackberries, blueberries

These berries contain "anthocyanins" and "proanthocyanidins" which reduce hemorrhoidal pain and swelling by toning and strengthening the hemorrhoid
veins. Drink at least one glass of this juice mixture each day.

Cantaloupe

Cantaloupes are one of the best foods you can eat. It has a good source of vitamins and minerals. It has a high beta-carotene level and has anti-clogging properties.

Red and Black Currant Berries

Currants are high in Vitamin C, rutin, and minerals. This makes their juice valuable in clearing hemorrhoids. This also has a small amount of the fatty acid GLA, which produce prostaglandin that control body pain.

This juice is also good for cleansing the liver and blood. Good liver function is necessary for maintaining a healthy colon, rectum and anus.

Drink 1 –2 glasses a day of red or black currant berries.

Pomegranate Juice

Although pomegranate juice may be hard to find, it is quite useful in reducing hemorrhoids, because of its strong astringency. Saturate a cotton ball with pomegranate juice and push it slightly into your rectum.

If you have pinworms, the tannins in pomegranate juice will help you get rid of them. You can also drink the juice. During the summer I have on occasion found pomegranate juice at a farmers market. It is slightly tart but it is easy to
drink. However, it's hard to drink more than a glass full without getting a stomach upset.

Oranges and bananas

Eat 2-3 oranges and 2 bananas a day. Oranges provide vitamin C, bioflavonoids, and fiber. Bananas provide minerals that help to strengthen tissue and have plenty of fiber. Bananas can also be steamed to give more relief and even
eliminate hemorrhoids. Steam two not quite ripe bananas with their peel until they are soft. Eat two in the morning and two in the evening.

Papaya

Papaya is an excellent fruit to eat. It has good mineral content, fiber, and has enzymes to digest protein.

These are the fruits and juices to use to for relieving hemorrhoids. Adding more vegetables to your eating habits is also important to get more fiber. These fruits, juices, and vegetables will help you keep regular and provide pain and inflammation relief for your hemorrhoid symptoms.

Heartburn, Indigestion and Ulcer Relief Using DGL

In the 1940's licorice was discovered to be useful in treating peptic ulcers. Unfortunately it had side effects that lead to high blood pressure, potassium loss, and fluid retention.

Researchers discovered that the ingredient in licorice that caused those side effects was "glycyrrhizin." They were able to remove 97% of this chemical and the result was a product call "deglycyrrhizinated" licorice, DGL. DGL maintained its healing properties but had no side effects.

DGL was first used to heal ulcers in the stomach and duodenum without suppressing stomach acids. DGL worked just as good as the drugs Zantac or Tagamet that are designed to suppress stomach acid.

As more people used DGL, they found they got relief from a variety of stomach issues - heartburn, acid reflux, indigestion, bloating, and gas. In addition, they found using DGL was better than using antacids or acid blockers.

DGL works by improving and restoring the integrity of the esophageal, stomach and duodenum lining. It does this by promoting mucus release and cell rebuilding. The mucus released provides gastrointestinal lining protection from acids and gives the lining time to rebuild and regenerated. The result is healing and strengthening of the affected tissue.

Here's how to use DGL. DGL comes in large tablets that you place in your mouth and allowed to melt. You can chew them slightly but not swallow them since it is your salvia that helps activate the DGL.

By allowing DGL to melt in your mouth the resulting liquid will now run along your esophagus and start the healing process where ever there is tissue inflammation or damage.

Use two tablets 3-4 times a day on an empty stomach. Do not use any water when you are taking the tablets. You can take the tablets at least an hour before you eat and an hour after you eat.

Although DGL provides relief for heartburn, acid reflux and other stomach disturbances it does not totally provide a cure. It does provide recover from damaged gastrointestinal lining as occurs with ulcers, but does not change the level of stomach acid.

In some cases Heartburn is caused by to little or to much stomach acid. When too little acid is causing heartburn or acid reflux it makes no sense to use antacids or acid blocking drugs which decrease your stomach acid even more. Low levels of stomach acid leads to serious illnesses.

Because so much is still unknown about the cause of acid reflux or heartburn, it is known that DGL can give you some acid reflux relief and in some case mild cases cure it.

Use DGL for mild or severe cases of heartburn or acid reflux and you will be surprised at the results you get.

Candida/Yeast

After years of working with clients with candida symptomology, I have found that until the yeast (candida albicans) is brought under control, the body cannot begin to heal with efficacy. Once again, we need to look at 'balance'. If the internal environment of the body is unbalanced, then that environment is an ideal situation for disease.

Friendly Bacteria:

Candida does have a purpose! When babies are born, their intestinal tracts have about 75% lacto bacillus acidophilus and about 25% e coli bacteria which are the 'non-friendly' bacteria. Yeast also exists in the intestines and plays the role of assisting in breaking down proteins. The problem occurs when these friendly and non-friendly bacteria get out of balance, thus allowing the yeast to proliferate.

So, what can cause an unbalance in friendly bacteria? All antibiotics kill friendly flora, as do cortisone-type drugs, oral contraceptives, and chemotherapeutic drugs. In addition, certain foods encourage the growth of Candida. Candida is a living micro-organism that thrives on all food products that are simple sugars, as well as all foods that turn to glucose (sugar) in the body. This includes most carbohydrates, such as refined white flours, rice, pasta, as well as products which contain yeast.

Symptoms:

The symptoms that can occur from systemic yeast are too numerous to mention; but here are just a few: extreme mood swings, irritability, depression, headaches, lethargy, gastritis, colitis, bloating, fluid in ears, itching, rashes, psoriasis, acne, spots in vision, blurred vision, nasal congestion and stuffiness, postnasal drip, cystitis, endometriosis, kidney or bladder infections, loss of appetite, overeating, insomnia, poor circulation, numbness and tingling, vaginal burning or itching, menstrual cramping, PMS, hay fever, asthma, food sensitivities, hives, loss of interest in sex, thrush, and colic.

Digestion: Proper digestion is the missing ingredient in many health programs. The role of digestion in controlling Candida is no exception. After eating a meal, the food begins to break down through enzymes produced by the body. Minerals in the bloodstream help the parietal glands in the stomach in making hydrochloric acid. This acidic reaction kills pathogens on the food and enables the protein and minerals to be further broken down by digestive juices. The small intestine walls do not have protective mucosa, so without this alkalizing mineral bath you would have burning and pain.

Once this process is complete, the food is in tiny pieces able to pass through the walls of the small intestines to be used as food energy at a cellular level. If this digestive process is working correctly you will be in good shape; given, of course, that your diet is rich in raw and organic foods.

However, most people slip up somewhere along the line. If you do not chew your food well to begin the digestive process, if your pancreas is not producing enough enzymes, and you don't make enough HCL then the pepsin cannot convert to pepsinogen in the stomach and protein digestion as well as mineral absorption is impaired. The body is then malnourished in spite of all your efforts to eat correctly.

Food that is in a state of partial digestion cannot cross the gut wall as nourishment. This can irritate the gut wall; or large partially digested food particles can cross through and circulate the blood stream in an unusable form. This state triggers a bodily response of defense.

Yeast is called upon to eat protein or starch that wasn't digested in the intestines. The more the yeast is fed, the more waste it makes. The waste from the overgrowth of yeast creates the problems which manifest as symptoms of disease.

Killing off the yeast helps….but is not the total answer. Good digestion is imperative. Food enzymes, particularly containing cellulase, which eats yeast, are an important part of any Candida program. There are several herbs which can get the yeast under control by killing it off. Here are a few: White pond lily, greasewood, purple loosestrife, pau d'arco, caprylic acid, oregano, and garlic.

Changing your diet: Avoid starchy foods, white flour, processed foods, and sugars. Packaged meats, canned goods, vinegar, yeast products, cakes, candy, mushrooms, alcohol, and peanuts are major foods to avoid. Your diet should consist mainly of fresh vegetables and organic meats in a balanced fashion. It is even best to avoid fruits and fruit juices for a short time while first doing a Candida/yeast cleanse.

After taking medications: Continuing on the digestive program of enzymes which contain cellulase is a must at all times; but particularly after a bout of antibiotics, or constant use of oral contraceptives. After all Candida/yeast programs, it is important to follow up with refloridation of the friendly bacteria in the colon.

Acidophilus, bifidophilus, and other strains of healthy bacteria are necessary. If the intestinal system is in a state of cleanliness, with good peristalsis; the friendly bacteria will eventually begin to repopulate on their own.

Candida can be kept in check.

Ginko Biloba - Helping Memory and Circulation

Ginko Biloba

Ginkgo Biloba is one of the oldest living tree species, dating back over 300 million years. Individual trees can live for over 1,000 years. Ginkgo Biliboa is the best selling herbal product in the world. It is an extract from the green leaves of the Ginkgo tree which is native to Asia, however, is grown worldwide. The active ingredients in the extract are the Ginkgoflavoneglycos, Bilobalide, and terpenelactones including ginkgolides A, B and C. In Asia, ginkgo tree extracts have been used for over 5,000 years to treat cardiovascular problems as well as lung disorders.

Ginkgo's most powerful effect is on the circulating system. Ginkgo flavenoids directly dilate the smallest segment of the circulating system, the micro-capillaries, which increase both blood circulation and oxygen levels in the brain as well as in other critical organ tissues. Ginkgo also prevents platelet aggregation or clumping inside the arterial walls. This increases arterial wall strength and flexibility and decreases the opportunity for the formation of arteriosclerostic plague.

Since ginkgo increases oxygen flow to the brain and enhances the brains uptake and utilization of glucose it also is being researched for its role in the senility, forgetfulness, headaches and Alzheimer's disease and its role in improving alertness, memory and mental performance. Recent studies indicate that some patients exhibiting the symptoms of these ailments enjoyed marginal improvement in cognitive abilities after using Ginko.

In addition to the benefits provided to the brain by Ginko, it has been shown that Ginko can also help reduce the frequency and intensity of depression.

Related to circulatory improvement, German researchers have also been studying ginkgo as a treatment for atheroclerotic peripheral vascular disease. This disease impairs walking and ginkgo has been shown to help blood flow to the legs allowing people to walk further with far less pain. Ginkgo is a highly important antioxidant shown to have a special affinity for scavenging the superoxide radicals.

Benefits

- Increases circulation to the brain and lower extremities
- Treats senile conditions such as Alzheimer's disease
- Treats loss of concentration and emotional fatigue in the elderly
- Treats hardening of the arteries
- Treats depression
- Treats allergies
- May treat tinnitus and vertigo
- May reduce vision loss due to aging
- May reduce symptoms associated with Raynaud's disease
- Possible assistance in the treatment of peripheral vascular disease

Ginseng

Ginseng is the most famous Chinese herb. It is the most widely recognized plant used in traditional medicine. Various forms of ginseng have been used in medicine for more than 7000 years. Several species grow around the world, and though some are preferred for specific benefits, all are considered to have similar properties as an effective general rejuvenator.

Ginseng is a slow growing perennial herb (reaches about 2 feet tall) native to the mountainous area of north eastern China, Korea and far eastern regions of Russia. The older the root, the greater the concentration of ginsenosides, the active chemical compounds, thus the more potent the ginseng becomes. Ginseng roots can live longer than hundreds of years. Ginseng has been cultivated extensively in China, Korea, and Japan, and Russia.

Ginseng starts flowering in fourth year, and the roots take 4-6 years to reach maturity. Ginseng is a protected herb in China and Russia: exporting ginseng seeds is banned in China, and harvesting wild ginseng is illegal in Russia. Natural white ginseng is often steam- processed to produce "red ginseng" with different, higher medicinal potency.

It is used to reduce the effects of stress, improve performance, boost energy levels, enhance memory, and stimulate the immune system. Oriental medicine has deemed ginseng a necessary element in all their best prescriptions, and regards it as prevention and a cure. It is said to remove both mental and bodily fatigue, cure pulmonary complaints, dissolve tumors and reduce the effects of age.

Ginseng is native to China, Russia, North Korea, Japan, and some areas of North America. It was first cultivated in the United States in the late 1800's. It is difficult to grow and takes 4-6 years to become mature enough to harvest. The roots are called Jin-chen, meaning 'like a man,' in reference to their resemblance to the shape of the human body.

Native North Americans considered it one of their most sacred herbs and add it to many herbal formulas to make them more potent. The roots can live for over 100 years.

Ginseng contains vitamins A, B-6 and the mineral Zinc, which aids in the production of thymic hormones, necessary for the functioning of the defense system. The main active ingredients of ginseng are the more than 25 saponin triterpenoid glycosides called "ginsenosides".

These steroid-like ingredients provide the adaptogenic properties that enable ginseng to balance and counter the effects of stress. The glycosides appear to act on the adrenal glands, helping to prevent adrenal hypertrophy and excess corticosteroid production in response to physical, chemical or biological stress.

Studies done in China showed that ginsenosides also increase protein synthesis and activity of neurotransmitters in the brain. Ginseng is used to restore memory, and enhance concentration and cognitive abilities, which may be impaired by improper blood supply to the brain.

Ginseng helps to maintain excellent body functions. Siberian ginseng has been shown to increase energy, stamina, and help the body resist viral infections and environmental toxins. Research has shown specific effects that support the central nervous system, liver function, lung function and circulatory system.

Animal studies have shown that ginseng extracts stimulate the production of interferons, increase natural killer cell activity, lower cholesterol and decrease triglyceride levels. Men have used the herb to improve sexual function and remedy impotence. Ginseng is believed to increase estrogen levels in women and is used to treat menopausal symptoms.

It is also used for diabetes, radiation and chemotherapy protection, colds, chest problems, to aid in sleep, and to stimulate the appetite.

Korean Red Ginseng is also known by the names Asian Ginseng, Asiatic Ginger, and Chinese Ginseng. Korean Red Ginseng is a deciduous perennial shrub whose fleshy root requires 4-6 years of cultivation to reach maturity.

Korean Red Ginseng is now used as a natural preventive, restorative remedy and valued for its adaptogenic properties. Korean Red Ginseng is considered most suitable for males and for older people. Used for centuries in China, Korean Red Ginseng was believed to be and anti-aging herb. By equalizing the system levels in the body, Korean Red Ginseng has been used to lower cholesterol, balance the metabolism, increase energy levels, and stimulate the immune system.

Korean White Ginseng is an adaptogen having yang properties and an arousing and stimulating metabolic effect on the central nervous system, brain, head, and blood vessels. It may benefit blood sugar levels, histamine levels, inflammation, stress levels, mental and physical abilities, impotency, anemia, artery hardening, depression, diabetes, ulcers, edema, immune and lung function, appetite, libido and may offer protection against radiation exposure and easement of cocaine withdrawal.

North American White Ginseng (Panax quinquefolium) is believed to give a cooling effect to the body. This cooling, energy giving, endurance enhancing factor is believed to be the most beneficial for our fast paced, stressful world.

Siberian ginseng is a distinct plant with different active chemical components. Prized for its ability to restore vigor, increase longevity, enhance overall health, and stimulate both a healthy appetite and a good memory, it is widely used in Russia to help the body adapt to stressful conditions and to enhance productivity.

Benefits
• reduce the effects of stress
• boost energy levels
• assists with mental and body fatigue

Gout

The name of the disease is not what concerns the person who treats the patient holistically, for they are looking at the die-ease in the patient, not the gout. Gout is a manifestation of the disease in the patient, treating the presenting symptoms with drugs for the inflammation and pain may well relieve the symptoms temporarily, but it's not treating the cause of the condition.

So what is the cause of gout? One might be told that some families have a predisposition to gout, and you may be told that some foods exacerbate the condition, and that's about all that can be done if you are treated conventionally, you will also be given some prescription drugs to alleviate your pain, and to reduce inflammation. If you do nothing else to correct the cause of your gout, then it's very unlikely you will see any improvement in your health.

You may say that since you have been taking a certain drug that you haven't had any gout attacks, and as far as you are concerned not much else matters. Unfortunately the prescription drugs have only palliated your condition, and with constant ingestion of anti-inflammatory drugs and pain killers your gouty condition will continue to develop behind the scenes and your general health will deteriorate as a result of the drugs you are taking.

Alternative medicine, depending on what modality you have chosen, would firstly want to overhaul your diet, for a diet rich in purine foods would certainly exacerbate the condition, and may even be solely responsible for your gout.

Foods high in purines and are therefore to be avoided: Meat gravies, stocks, organ meats, shellfish, anchovies, sardines, herrings, mussels, mushrooms and asparagus. Alcohol, particularly beer is high in purines, and for that reason must be avoided. Any alcohol taken should be followed by copius amounts of water to avoid dehydration and consequent uric acid build-up.

Meat, white flour, sugar, poultry, dried beans, fish, oatmeal, cauliflower, spinach and peas are moderately high in purines, and may need to be avoided.

The ideal diet should contain lots of organic fresh fruit, vegetables, whole grains, and a very important dietary addition is wheatgrass. Fruits, vegetables and juices assist the excretion of uric acid, and foods that neutralize uric acid are strawberries, cherries, and celery juice, also drink lots of filtered water. Many people have found that the addition of cherry juice to their diet has prevented further gout attacks.

You may be given herbs or homeopathic remedies for your condition; however a change in your dietary habits may be all that is needed to improve your health. What a simple answer to what could remain a lifetime problem if you may no effort to change your eating habits. If you wish to rid yourself of your gout, alternative medicine can certainly help you.

Health Care for Globe Trotters

Motion sickness:

Almost everybody is susceptible to motion sickness. Fatigue, giddiness, deprivation of sleep, nausea and vomiting are the main unwelcome symptoms of motion sickness. Avoid consuming alcohol, pain killers, spicy foods, fried foods and junk foods during traveling. Try to relax and chose a window seat. Do not read or talk. Or watch someone who is motion sick.

Eat light food. Include pomegranate, ginger and curds in your diet while traveling. Rinse your mouth and wash your face with cold water as soon as you take your food.

Diarrhea:

Though travelers' diarrhea is mild inconvenience to a traveler, it may at times be life threatening too. Upsets in digestive system frequently occur in travelers due to stress, time zone changes, irregular meal times and new foods. But serious diarrhea during traveling is caused by bacteria, viruses or parasitic infections. The best way out is to take ample precautionary measures.

Wash your hands frequently. Use sanitizing liquids, hand washes or gels which cleanse the hands without water. Always use disposable hygienically packed tissue papers than towels. Avoid street, roadside foods, buffet meals. Select food which is well cooked and served hot. Thick-skinned fruits which you can peel yourself are usually safe. Avoid raw or undercooked meat, fish, uncooked vegetables, salads.

Be care full with unpasteurized milk and milk products. Always use sealed mineral water, canned juices and beverages. Never use ice cubes or unsealed bottled beverages. Bottled Beer, wine and hot coffee or tea are safe. Drink from original containers or clean glasses.

If you get mild diarrhea eat light, soft and semi solid foods like idli, soups etc which are easily digestible. Avoid heavy, spicy and non vegetarian foods. Drink plenty of fruit juices.(canned or hygienically packed.). Keep yourself well hydrated. Consult a doctor immediately if diarrhea leads to dehydration.

Constipation:

People often become constipated when traveling because their normal diet and daily routines are disrupted. Drink plenty of water and consume food which are rich in fibers to avoid constipation.

Try to adhere to routine food timings .Drink a big glass of water every day morning. Avoid frequent consumption of tea or coffee. Taking two thriphala tablets with warm water before going to bed helps to normalize bowel movements. These tablets should be avoided during pregnancy.

Tired feet

Even healthy people can get blood clots in their legs after long hours of traveling. Try to walk every now and then. Drink water, stretch your calf muscles while you're sitting and wear support stockings.

Foot bath for tired feet: Massage your foot with little coconut oil and soak them in warm water. You can add few drops of lavender oil or peppermint oil or sandal wood oil to warm water. After a foot bath rub your foot. Relax after a foot bath.

Prevention of Malaria:

To prevent mosquito bites and malaria wear mosquito repellent .Stay indoors between dusk and dawn. The malaria spreading mosquitoes generally feed at this time. Apply mosquito repellent, to your clothes and bedding. Wear socks, long pants, and long-sleeve shirts when outdoors. Use a mosquito net while sleeping. Stay in air-conditioned, screened accommodation.

Jet lag

To avoid jet lag get plenty of sleep before you leave. Don't drink a lot of alcohol while on flight. Eat well-balanced meals and avoid over eating. Exercise as much as you can on your trip. Get used to a new time zone by going along with the local meal and bedtime schedules.

Accidents:

Do not drive in unfamiliar places where you know less about that regional language, road conditions, rules of the road, condition of the vehicles. Etc. Choose your transportation carefully. Check the security, life saving facilities provided in the transport. Choose the cab with seat belts, hotels with fire escape and ferries with life preservers. Never swim in unknown rivers or seas when you are not familiar with sea currents and waves.

Sex:

Have a safe sex when you are with unfamiliar new partners. Alcohol, drugs and sex are dangerous combination

Immunization:

Get immunized with vaccines before traveling. Avoid animal bites and saliva. If you are bitten by dog wash the wound immediately with soap and water.

Travel during pregnancy:

If you chose to travel during pregnancy the second trimester (weeks 14 to 27) is the best time. Before traveling take the opinion of your consulting doctor and provide him the sufficient details about the places you are visiting, mode of transport etc.

Tips for older travelers

See your doctor for a checkup and discuss your fitness .See your dentist and ophthalmologist. Keep a spare pair of glasses, any medications you need in a small medical kit. Organize travel health insurance with pre-existing illness cover if needed. Make sure it covers emergency evacuation. Make sure routine immunizations are done before traveling.

Consider your back - use luggage with built in wheels. Take clothes and hats to suit the climate.

Other safety precautions:

Check with the regional office or through internet the situation of places you are planning to visit. The destination places must be free from riots, terrorism, floods or other calamities.

Mental tensions:

Preparations for traveling lead to worry and tensions. Here are few relaxing tips before and during traveling.

1.   Close your eyes , take five deep breaths through your nose and pay attention only to your breathing while doing this.

2.   Taking a hot shower relaxes your muscles and the break from more stressful activities helps too.

3.   Laugh. Laughing helps to relax. Find people who can make you laugh and make your moments lighter..

4.   Listen to relaxing music.

5.   Take a walk.

6.   Get a hug.

A visit to your family physician and some thought and planning ahead make your trip more successful and memorable. We wish you a rewarding, memorable, safe and healthy trip.

Health Solutions with Ashwagandha

Also known as Winter Cherry and Indian Ginseng, Ashwagandha is one of the most valuable herbs in the Ayurvedic medical system, dating back more than 3,000 years. Its Sanskrit name Ashwagandha literally means 'that which has the smell of a horse', so named because it is said to give the strength and vitality of a horse. Ashwagandha is specific for a wide range of conditions including arthritic inflammation, anxiety, insomnia, respiratory disorders, nervous disorders, gynecological disorders, male infertility and impotence.

It is a herb that enhances resistance to stress, increases stamina and promotes general well-being. Many Western herbalists refer to this herb as "Ayurvedic ginseng" because of its reputation for increasing energy, strength, and stamina, and for its ability to relieve stress.

Modern research has found several types of alkaloids in it of which somniferin and withaniol are responsible for its multiple actions. The roots of the plant have been reported to have Alkaloids, Withanolides and many Glycosides.

According to the Ayurvedic system, Ashwagandha is the best herb for balancing Vata in the body. Vata governs all movement in the body, including the movement of nerve impulses throughout the nervous system.

When the root is taken as a milk decoction and sweetened with honey or raw sugar, it is used to inhibit ageing and build up strength by catalysing the anabolic processes in the body.

Ashwagandha is also a proven immune-modulator, antioxidant and hormone precursor which tends to regulate important physiological functions. Research has shown that it can protect the activity of immune cells that are exposed to chemicals that would otherwise inhibit their normal function.

The antitumor activity of Withania somnifera is known and that it also enhances the effects of radiation in chemotherapy

Ashwagandha for Sexual Debility: Ashwagandha has an affinity for the reproductive system in both men and women. It is the main rejuvenative of masculine energy used in Ayurveda, improving the quality of reproductive tissues and increasing sexual potency. It has also been used to increase libido and potency, for it is said to bestow upon its user the vitality and strength of a horse.

It is often added in herbal supplements that are reputed to improve sexual desire and function. Ashwagandha has also been helping women boost their desire for sex. Long considered India's most potent sex-enhancing plant, the country's women have used Ashwagandha for years to rev up their sex drives

Ashwagandha For Stress: Ashwagandha is considered as one of the best remedies for stress. While most adaptogens primarily work by helping the body to mobilize and maintain the physiological response to stress, Ashwagandha appears to work first and foremost by reducing the stress-related excesses of the alarmed nervous system.

It improves the body's ability to maintain physical effort and helps the body adapt to various types of stress. It has also been reported to enhance mental function and memory. It acts to calm the mind and promote sound, restful sleep.

Ashwagandha as a Anti-Inflammatory Agent: Ashwagandha is an adaptogen that contains several active phytochemicals known as glycowithanolides, which research has shown may relax smooth muscles.

As a natural anti-inflammatory agent, ashwagandha may help to reduce the discomfort associated with arthritis.

Forty-two patients with osteoarthritis were randomly placed in two groups--one receiving ashwagandha, one a placebo. After three months, pain and disability were markedly reduced in the ashwagandha group.

Ashwagandha for Weak Memory: Ashwagandha is a medhya rasayana, helping to enhance mental ability and performance. It helps support memory and problem-solving skills and enhances the coordinated functioning of all aspects of the brain. It corrects loss of memory arising out of long term stress, illness and overwork.

Ashwagandha is also used for High Blood Pressure, as an Immune-Modulator and an AntiOxidant.

Hemorrhoids Treatment

Over 150 million of the living people in America today will experience some kind of hemorrhoids by the age of 50. Most will do nothing about it. Only 500,000 are expected to seek help this year. It is a crazy statistic, because for most people, hemorrhoids can be prevented and cured by making a few simple changes to lifestyle, diet and the use of an anti-inflammatory gel/cream.

There are 2 types of hemorrhoids, internal and external, both of which left unchecked can lead to more severe cases, and ultimately surgery. But that is if you do nothing about it. And there is not much to look forward to if you need surgery. Surgery is an excruciatingly painful experience, especially post-op.

Many patients have reported days, if not weeks of pain during the healing period after surgery. You see the outer rectum is one of the most sensitive parts of the body, and the most prevalent surgeries involve burning off hemorrhoids, or banding (tying a band around the affected area until it drops off) which leaves the area extremely tender, and when the patient needs to have a bowel movement, the pain can be even more excruciating than the hemorrhoids ever were.

But that is what happens if you do NOT attend to your hemorrhoids early. And considering that one of the major causes of hemorrhoids is from straining during bowel movements due to poor diet/lifestyle, and then there really is no reason that most sufferers can't avoid getting more/worse hemorrhoids.

That is, most people strain during a bowel movement because the stool (feces) has become hard and require a lot of pushing and straining. Simple changes to diet and lifestyle can improve regularity and reduce painful 'straining' bowel movements, and thus wipe-out the cause of hemorrhoids.

This is where the health of your colon kicks in. The colon (large intestine) can hold anywhere between 6-40lbs of fecal matter in the average adult. People who experience regular bowel movements (at least once daily), typically have a lot less of this fecal matter in their system, and quite obviously people who are less 'regular' have a lot more in their system. The colon, the last major part of the digestive system, actually draws a lot of water out of the fecal matter (stool) before it reaches the rectum. If the stool spends too much time in the colon, or if your diet is missing some key foods, then too much water is drawn out of the stool, and this is when you experience a hard bowel movement that requires straining and pushing....resulting in hemorrhoids.

There is much debate about what causes the stool to spend more time in the colon and thus become harder, but most agree that a clean and clear colon will assist in helping the stool to move freely and smoothly through the intestine. Couple this diet rich in water and fiber (which assists in making the stool softer and easier to pass) and you're on the right path towards reducing the cause of hemorrhoids.

Exercise is another major factor in improving you inner health. Many experts believe that exercise assists in speeding up our metabolic rate which actually sees our digestive system work quick, thus resulting in 'regularity' and less fecal matter sitting virtually idle in the digestive system (colon).

So if you have a diet that incorporates a lot of fiber (whole meal breads/cereal and fruits), you drink ample water (6-8 glasses daily) and you partake in regular exercise, then you could well be on your way towards improving your inner health, improving your bowel-movement regularity and reducing your hemorrhoids.

And for many people who are already 'dealing' with hemorrhoids, the use of an anti-inflammatory cream/gel can be the first step in helping to cure, and rid themselves of their hemorrhoids. Poor diet, laziness and lack of hydrating fluids are CAUSES of hemorrhoids, so making improvements in these areas will probably help to ease the current hemorrhoids, but will NOT FULLY CURE the sufferer.

The use of an anti-inflammatory will assist here (in most cases) by soothing the affected area, and also helping with circulation in the rectum area. These products act as a kind of decongestant in the rectum by reducing the swelling, which naturally brings with it better blood circulation in the veins, which in turn helps to diminish the size and existence of the hemorrhoids.